Essential Oils

Relieve Stress, Enhance Your Beauty, Improve Your Mood, Control Your Appetite, and More - All Naturally

By Jana Ceesay

Legal & Disclaimer

The information contained in this book and its contents is not designed to replace or take the place of any form of medical or professional advice; and is not meant to replace the need for independent medical, financial, legal or other professional advice or services, as may be required. The content and information in this book have been provided for educational and entertainment purposes only.

The content and information contained in this book has been compiled from sources deemed reliable, and it is accurate to the best of the Author's knowledge, information and belief. However, the Author cannot guarantee its accuracy and validity and cannot be held liable for any errors and/or omissions. Further, changes are periodically made to this book as and when needed. Where appropriate and/or necessary, you must consult a professional (including but not limited to your doctor, attorney, financial advisor or such other professional advisor) before using any of the suggested remedies, techniques, or information in this book.

Upon using the contents and information contained in this book, you agree to hold harmless the Author from and against any damages, costs, and expenses, including any legal fees potentially resulting from the application of any of the information provided by this book. This disclaimer applies to any loss, damages or injury caused by the use and application, whether directly or indirectly, of any advice or information presented, whether for breach of contract, tort, negligence, personal injury, criminal intent, or under any other cause of action.

You agree to accept all risks of using the information presented inside this book.

You agree that by continuing to read this book, where appropriate and/or necessary, you shall consult a professional (including but not limited to your doctor, attorney, or financial advisor or such other advisor as needed) before using any of the suggested remedies, techniques, or information in this book.

Table of Contents

Introduction 5

Chapter 1: Benefits of Aromatherapy 9

Chapter 2: Essential Oils for Weight Loss 11

Chapter 3: Essential Oils for Mental Health................13

Chapter 4: How Essential Oils are Used 15

   1.   As an Air Purifier 15

   2.   Insect Repellant 16

   3.   To Remove Odors from Your Environment.........16

   4.   For Home Cleanliness 16

   5.   In Cooking 17

   6.   To Clean Sportswear and Everyday Laundry 17

Chapter 5: Essential oil for Beauty 18

   A Refreshing Start 19

   Cleansing pastes recipes 19

   Exfoliating scrubs 21

   Steam treatments for your face..................................22

   Facial oil recipes 24

   Away with Wrinkles 27

   Conclusion 30

Introduction

Essential oil concentrated essences extracted from certain species of flowers, fruit, grasses, roots, resins, leaves and trees have been valued since ancient times for their therapeutic properties. There are about 300 different essential oils manufactured today. Many of these oils are used as ingredients in modern medicine. By using essential oils in your everyday life, you can avoid chemical-based preparations that can have adverse health effects. Natural essential oils can supplement almost any therapeutic treatment, from stress relief to energizing. Essential oils can be used to naturally promote your health and overall well-being while avoiding harsh side-effects that artificial chemicals can cause. Essential oils also have practical uses outside of health, as they can be used around your household to cleanse, purify the air, and refresh.

History

Essential oils are mankind's first medicines. Egyptian hieroglyphics found on tomb walls prove that essential oils were used in the embalming process, in healing ceremonies, religious ceremonies, in cosmetics, and for various medicinal purposes. Recipes for these oils and their uses were first found on the Ebers Papyrus, a medical scroll over 870 feet long. The scroll had over 800 herbal preparations, essential oil recipes and remedies. Other ancient scrolls describe treating 81 different diseases using myrrh and honey. Myrrh essential oil is still known for its ability to clear up infections of the skin and throat.

When King Tut's tomb was opened in 1922, there were more than 50 alabaster jars used for essential oils. The oils were gone, and only traces were left behind. Some stores of gold were undisturbed, and it is assumed that the grave robbers valued the essential oils above gold.

Ancient Chinese medical practitioners passed down their knowledge of essential oils used for curing common illnesses and calming down "disturbed minds." They dip their acupuncture needles in essential oils for a deeper sense of healing.

Practitioners from India used herbs and aromatic plants in their Ayurvedic medicinal system for thousands of years. They distilled essential oils to use in massage therapy and left recipes for essential oils that provide medical enhancements.

The Greeks followed the ways of the Egyptians and the most well-known physician of that time, Hippocrates, was a firm believer in holistic medicine and aromatherapy massage. It is believed that Hippocrates stopped a plague in Athens by using essential oils. In ancient Greece, Dioscorides wrote a book that described methods still used by aromatherapists today. Essential oils were extensively used to purify public buildings in opening ceremonies and were essential elements in steam baths.

The Arabian empire drew on the Greek and Roman experiences and uses of essential oils. The Persian physician Avicenna was credited with perfecting the distillation process of essential oils in 1037 AD.

Arabian traders used frankincense essential oil as a commodity. Frankincense was and is very expensive and was often valued more than gold.

During the Black Plague of the 17th century, essential oils, specifically lavender, was spread over the floors of the castles and individuals fastened bunches of lavender to their wrists to protect themselves. Lavender is a known insect repellent and wards off mosquitos. Those who wore lavender may have escaped the Black Plague since mosquitos were culprits in spreading Black Plague. Lavender stops mosquitos from biting.

By the late 1800s, the active elements of natural remedies were isolated, and essential oils began their modern comeback. Dr. Rene-Maurice Gattefosse, Ph.D., a French chemist, began studying essential oils in 1907. In 1910, Dr. Gattefosse was terribly burned in a laboratory accident. He plunged his hands into a vat of lavender, and the lavender solution stopped the gasification of the tissue. He began studying essential oils and their properties in earnest and is now credited with being the father of aromatherapy.

Essential oils were used during World War I by Dr. Monciere. He used essential oils for their wound-healing and antibacterial properties. He also developed different types of aromatic ointments to ease the pain and suffering among the soldiers.

Dr. Jean Valnet, a colleague of Dr. Gattefosse, practiced medicine in Tonkin, China during WWII. Dr. Valnet exhausted his supply of antibiotics and began using therapeutic-grade essential oils on soldiers' injuries. To his glee and surprise, these essential oils actually combated and counteracted infection. He saved the lives of numerous soldiers who might have otherwise died of wound infection and inflammation. The work of Dr. Valnet was carried on by two of his students who further broke down and wrote about the anti-viral, antibacterial, antifungal and antiseptic properties of essential oils.

The 1980s led to the rediscovery of essential oils in the United States. The role that essential oils play in combating present-day diseases is being researched and believers are using essential oils more than ever.

Today there are numerous massage clinics that blend their own essential oils and deeply believe in the healing power of massage and essential oil application.

Elements

Essential oils are those wonderful, but volatile or somewhat unpredictable liquids made naturally in plants. Technically, essential oils are not oils at all but highly concentrated plant components. The determining factors of the strength and beneficial values of an essential oil is in its chemical and organic compounds. These compounds come about due to a number of factors. These features include the stems, flowers, bark or root of the plant where the oil is produced, soil conditions, organic or chemical fertilizers, climate, altitude harvest season, geographic regions and distillation processes.

Chapter 1: Benefits of Aromatherapy

The survival of aromatherapy is attributed to all the benefits of essential oils. It is not a medically prescribed solution, but the use of essential oils has proven to be very helpful for a variety of concerns. In this chapter, you will learn more about how aromatherapy will be beneficial to your mental and physical health.

The human mind and body are prone to many different ailments at any point in time. This is why it's important to take extra care and provide it with the nurture it needs. Aromatherapy is one of the best methods of practicing self-care. It can be used to address a variety of issues without harming the body or being heavy on your wallets.

- Aromatherapy is very helpful in relieving stress, anxiety, depression, and such mental concerns.
- The essential oils are a natural alternative to other substances that are loaded with harmful chemicals or other additives.
- The natural alternatives are much more affordable methods and potent for healing.
- Topical application through massages improves blood circulation throughout the body.
- The oils can help in the relaxation of the muscles and relieving tension from the body.

- Essential oils boost the immune system and help in fighting diseases.
- The oils can be used internally as well as externally.
- The benefits of aromatherapy are long term and not just a quick fix.
- It can be used to address skin issues like eczema.

- Aromatherapy helps in relieving pain or aches in the joints or any body parts.

- Certain essential oils can also work as disinfectants and have anti-bacterial, anti-fungal properties.

- The functioning of the various organs can also be improved with the help of aromatherapy.

- Essential oils are also good for improving sexual performance.

- Diffusion of some essential oils helps to cleanse the air and also get rid of unpleasant odors from the surroundings.

- Essential oils can help improve the texture and appearance of skin and hair.

These points as mentioned above are just the overall benefits of using essential oils in aromatherapy. Respectively, each essential oil has its own unique set of properties that can be beneficial for many different concerns you may have. You will learn more about these further on.

Chapter 2: Essential Oils for Weight Loss

Eating unhealthy food and irregular food habits will usually lead to excessive weight gain. Obesity has become an increasingly imminent disease, especially amongst youth. Your lifestyle habits affect your eating habits, and thus your body. All the junk food, sugar-laden food, and eating out mean that you don't take in actual nutrition. If you don't pay enough attention to eating regular meals and healthy wholesome foods, you will inevitably gain more weight than is healthy for your body. There are other forms of diseases associated with excess weight as well. To deal with these issues, you can try using aromatherapy and essential oils. Essential oils can be used in different ways to help with weight loss. You can use them to massage onto the skin or even inhale the essential oils. Certain essential oils can also be consumed internally to aid in improving digestion and losing weight. They can help you to reduce stress-related eating and also flush out toxins.

- **Peppermint essential oil** contains Vitamin C as well as Omega-3 fatty acids. It will help you to lose weight as the diffusion of this prevents unhealthy hunger cravings and makes you feel more satiated for a longer time.

- You can improve digestion with the help of **Ginger essential oil.** It also helps in energizing your body.

- Unhealthy diets cause a lot of toxin build-up in the body. **A lemon essential oil** can be used for detoxification and also improves digestion. The oil also improves a person's appetite healthily. It can be consumed, inhaled, and massaged, so you can utilize it in your preferred way.

- Running a bath with certain essential oils helps to boost the process of fat burning. One fat burning blend can be made with **cypress, orange, and juniper.** Another blend for this purpose is **Lemon, Coconut, Peppermint, and Grapefruit** essential oils. Adding apple cider vinegar to hot water with **Rosemary, Lemon, and Orange** essential oils also helps.

- If you suffer from bloating, it is usually due to water retention. **Grapefruit essential oil** is effective in dealing with this concern. You can drink some warm water with a few drops of this oil to aid in reducing bloating and also for flushing out toxins.

- Unhealthy food cravings are often caused by stress. Stress eating results in a lot of weight gain. You can inhale or massage some **Bergamot essential oil** to reduce stress. It also helps in lowering levels of LDL cholesterol in the body.

- Add some **cinnamon essential oil** into your water to improve the functioning of the digestive system and boost your metabolism. This oil increases the rate of sugar breakdown and prevents fats from storing in the body.

- It is important to curb over-eating habits, and this can be done with the help of **sandalwood essential oil**. It promotes relaxation and pushes away stressful emotions. The oil can be diffused in the surroundings or even consumed with some water.

- Cellulite in the body can be dealt with by massaging a blend **of Cedarwood and cypress essential oils** with some carrier oil — these help in improving the blood circulation around the body.

- Another blend used for treating cellulite is created by mixing **juniper, fennel, and Geranium essential oils.**

Chapter 3: Essential Oils for Mental Health

In our daily lives, we put a lot of pressure on our physical as well as our mental health. These days, most people suffer from stress or anxiety. There is always so much to do, so little time and everyone is struggling to achieve success. Achieving success should never come at the price of your inner peace. Essential oils will help you in relieving stress and anxiety and help in promoting emotional well-being. Massages with essential oils are very helpful to relieve pain or aches in the body and also get rid of stress and tension. Diffusion of different oils benefits in many ways, like alleviation of negative emotions. Addressing mental issues regularly is important to avoid culmination of more serious problems. The olfactory senses can affect the brain and change emotions with the use of aromatherapy. Use them to your benefit to see better emotional health.

- **Anxiety can be relieved with the help of** Clary Sage, Frankincense, and Bergamot essential oil.

- **For a relaxing blend, you can mix** Clary Sage with Lavender and Marjoram.

- If you have insomnia, try mixing **Chamomile with Bergamot** essential oil and diffuse it in the room before sleeping.

- If you suffer from frequent mood swings, try diffusing some **orange essential oil** in your room to help balance your emotions. Another oil good for regulating mood swings is **Ylang-Ylang essential oil.**

- Depression is emerging as a more common mental ailment these days. You can alleviate feelings associated with this condition by using a blend of **sandalwood, orange, and Rose essential oils**.

- Make a massage oil with a blend of **cypress and grapefruit essential oil** and add **basil** to it. It works as an energizing element, which will relieve fatigue.

- Sometimes, you need help to deal with feelings of anger and resentment against the people around us. You can try using **Rosemary, Ylang-Ylang, and Jasmine essential oils** to make you feel calmer. Aggressive behavior will also be improved with the diffusion of **Chamomile, Lemon, and Rosemary essential oils.**

- Add **sandalwood and Rose essential oils** to a warm bath to alleviate sad feelings.

- Grief is an inevitable emotion in certain emotions. To feel better, try a blend of **Chamomile, Neroli, and Rose essential oils**.

- Pour some **Jasmine and Ylang-Ylang essential oils** in a warm bath to relax at the end of the day.

- To alleviate anxiety, draw a warm bath and add drops of **Vetiver, Rose, and Lavender essential oils.**

- Panic attacks can be very hard to deal with sometimes. Try a blend of **Geranium with juniper and Neroli essential oils** and inhale it once in a while. It will help you remain calm and relax.

- **Fatigue can be relieved essential oils like** Peppermint, Clove, Ginger and Jasmine essential oils.

- Use a diffuser with **Cypress and Grapefruit essential oils** to boost feelings of confidence.

- Infuse some **Jasmine and Rose** essential oils around you if you suffer from feelings of jealousy quite often. It can be an unhealthy emotion that affects your relationships and well-being.

Chapter 4: How Essential Oils are Used

Essential oils have actually been in use since centuries ago, and even after many years of scientific medicine being used, people still want to explore the various uses they can put essential oils to. For one, it is gratifying to know that whether you are using the essential oil personally, or you are using them on your child, you are using something natural. It is rare that natural products cause you side effects, and so essential oils continue to be very popular even amongst the pharmacologically inclined.

Generations over the years have used essential oils extensively for aromatherapy, and people of diverse cultural backgrounds have been using them for their medicinal value. In fact, whereas essential oils were, for some time, not wholly embraced within the science fraternity, today scientists are exploring the possibility of deriving modern medicine from the same plants the essential oils come. As days go by, scientists maintain hope that one of these days they are going to discover a cure for severe ailments such as seizure, stroke, cancer, and more.

Natural Essential Oils are Plentiful

Any idea how many of these much sought-after essential oils there are? There are hundreds! This is significant considering that almost every one of them has a health benefit in addition to the aspect of releasing nice, pleasant scents. They can give even better fragrances and offer better health benefits when they are used in combination with one another to create sophisticated blends.

Diverse Uses of Essential Oils

1.   As an Air Purifier

Who does not like to be in an environment that smells nice and fresh? You can successfully transform your home using essential oils, so that everyone in the house feels refreshed and comfortable. For instance, lemongrass and cinnamon

15

essential oil diffused into your room is known to fight bacteria in the air. Orange, lemon, and grapefruit essential oil are antimicrobial and fight airborne germs. Not only will people in your house enjoy the pleasant, refreshing air, but they will also be breathing air that has been cleared of unhealthy microbes.

2. **Insect Repellant**

How great it is that you can use natural essential oils as mosquito repellants, and not only will you be using substance that is pleasant, and safe for everyone to inhale, but you will also be repelling insects that are nuisance to the family. Mix together a drop of lemongrass oil, one of citronella oil, and another of the eucalyptus oil, then add a teaspoon of natural coconut oil to the mix. With this rich but easy to make essential oil blend, you will have made yourself a natural bug spray, which you can also rub onto skin that is irritated or itchy from a mosquito or other insect bite.

3. **To Remove Odors from Your Environment**

Here, you only need to take around 5 to 10 drops of whatever essential oil you choose, and then you put it in your garbage container. The essential oil can also do great when used to give fragrance to your vacuum bag. Mix your favorite air purifying oils with a bit of water in a spray bottle, then mist any areas of your home that need refreshing.

4. **For Home Cleanliness**

You can make an all-purpose cleaner from essential oils, and one thing that makes such a cleaner desirable is the fact that it is not only safe for you and your family members to use, but it is also environmentally friendly. A good example is the recipe that has the tree oil and lemon oils combined in proportions of 3 drops each, and then mixed with a couple of ounces of water. Once you have made this potent essential oil blend, you can spray a little of it on your kitchen counters, in the living room counters, and such other places, and you will effectively be disinfecting those places.

5.   In Cooking

Even though essential oils can be totally natural and organic, take care to research each oil before you attempt to ingest it. While most are harmless, some are definitely harmful if consumed. However, some oils can be used to enhance the flavor and aroma of your cooking. For example, you can mix in some nice smelling essential oils when baking sweets, such as peppermint oil, coconut oil, lavender, or lemon.

6.   To Clean Sportswear and Everyday Laundry

You can make a great garment cleaner from essential oils. For example, you can combine 2 drops of tea tree oil, 2 drops of lemon essential oil, and a single quart of water. If you then add to the mix 4 tablespoonfuls of baking soda, you will have made yourself an effective garment cleaner that will rid your sportswear of dirt and sweat, and leave your garments smelling wonderful. You can make your regular laundry smell even better by adding around 10 to 20 drops of your choice essential oil to the wash or rinse. Or enhance laundry even after drying by using a spray bottle to mist articles of clothing with a few drops of your favorite oil mixed with a bit of water.

Chapter 5: Essential oil for Beauty

The most common use of aromatherapy or essential oils is usually for beautification purposes all over the world. These are used in wellness centers or spas to help in relaxation and treating the body. The essential oils are a much safer alternative compared to using commercial skin care products, which have chemicals and harmful additives. All the heat applied on hair with straighteners and blow-dryers also has an adverse effect on the quality of hair. What you eat and your other habits will also determine the amount of hair you lose or the general health of your hair. Various oils can be used in different manners to treat hair and skin concerns. The natural approach results in long-term benefits instead of the harmful cosmetic application. Essential oils help in improving your inner health and not just what happens on the outside. You will soon see that your skin becomes clearer with fading marks and brighter complexion. Your hair will also grow longer and shinier with the help of the proper essential oils.

Initially only vegetable oils we used until the maceration method was invented that allowed for flowers and herbs to be added to the oils. Later as distillation was invented, essential oils became readily available. Any natural oil applied to the skin can leave a gleam that no other artificial substance can reproduce. When natural essential oils are applied to the skin regularly, it rejuvenates the skin and gives it a healthy glow.

You are faced with a large variety of essential oils to choose from in your beauty regimen and that includes both base oils (carrier oils) and essential oils. Not only should your beauty products make you look and feel great, but they should also feed and moisturize the skin. Remember that these oils are fragrant, so you have to make sure that the amount of oil you use appeals to your sense of smell as well. Essential oils are a delightful way for pampering your body and you can rest assured that these natural products will be good for your body, mind and spirit.

A Refreshing Start

We all wash our faces and bodies, and most of us use soaps or other specialty cleansers that fill the isles of our local stores. Making your own soaps and body washes are not only fun, but will also save you a lot of money in the long run. And by making your own products you can tweak the recipes to suit your own needs. Have fun experimenting to get the right properties and fragrances to suit every person in your family's needs. Another thing to remember is that everybody has different skin types. To compound the problem, remember that our skins have different needs as the seasons change. For this reason it makes sense to create your own cleansers to suit you for your age, skin type, skin needs and weather.

You might need a cleanser to remove makeup, grime, sweat or just a build-up of toxins.

All nut oils and vegetable oils will clean the skin while feeding and nourishing it at the same time. Ancient romans rubbed oils into the skin and scraped off the dirt and oil with a stick called a strigil before having a bath.

Select your base oils according to your skin type. Heavy oils like wheat germ oil or avocado oil work well on dry skin or on skin problems like eczema. For oily skin opt for lighter oils like almond oil or sunflower oil.

The best essential oils to use for cleansing the skin include: Chamomile, Clary Sage, Geranium Lemon, Lime, Lavender, Sage, Thyme and Rosemary.

Cleansing pastes recipes

- 150 ml Almond Oil

- 180 g finely ground Almonds

- 75 ml Distilled Water

- 75 ml Cider Vinegar

- 2 Drops of Chamomile Essential Oil

- 2 Drops of Geranium Essential Oil

- 2 Drops of Sage Essential Oil

- 2 Drops of Thyme Essential Oil

Blend all ingredients well for about 60 seconds. Add the essential oils and blend for another 60 seconds. Store the paste in an airtight container.

Luxurious Cleansing Cream

- 2 Drops of Clary Sage Essential Oil

- 2 Drops of Lemon Essential Oil

- 100 ml Distilled Water

- 15 g Beeswax

- 30 g Lanolin Hydrous

- 25 ml Avocado Oil

- 25 ml Grape Seed Oil

Melt the beeswax in a double boiler (a glass top part works best). Add the lanolin, almond, avocado and grape seed oils. Stir well. Stir after removing from heat. Use a whisk to mix the ingredients, while slowly adding the distilled water. Store in an airtight jar and use this cleanser on dry skin to rejuvenate and feed the skin.

Exfoliating scrubs

Exfoliating means cleaning the skin with an abrasive ingredient to scrub away dirt and dead skin cells. Oatmeal, sugar, even nuts like almonds or hazel nuts can be used as exfoliators. All you need to do is to process them in a food processor to a fine, but gritty consistency. It should look and feel like course sand. Oatmeal is an ingredient used in many commercial body cleaning and hair products. If you combine oatmeal with almonds you will have a scrub that will work very well on the face as well as other body parts.

Quick scrub for oily skin

- ¼ teaspoon salt

- ½ teaspoon cider vinegar

- 1 drop of Basil Essential Oil

- 1 teaspoon oatmeal

- 1 teaspoon ground almonds

Add the oatmeal and almonds after mixing the first ingredients well. Dampen your face and use your fingers to scrub the skin in small circular movements. Rinse your face twice with clean water and pat dry with a clean towel.

Deep clean scrub

- 1 teaspoon ground almonds

- ½ teaspoon almond oil

- 1 drop of Lemon Essential Oil

Dampen your face and apply the scrub. Let it sit for half a minute. Use your hands and gently massage the entire face to work the scrub into the pores of your skin. Rinse with clean cool water three times. Pat the skin dry with a clean towel.

Steam treatments for your face

Caution: Do not use this type of treatment on sensitive skin, sunburnt skin or if you have broken veins on the skin.

This forces grime, dirt and toxins out of the pores. Home steaming is very easy. All you need is a large bowl, boiling water, a towel and the recipe ingredients.

Pour the boiling water into the bowl. Add the essential oil or oils into the water. Hold your head about 18-20 inches from the surface of the water and place a towel over your head to form a tent around the bowl. Close your eyes and let the steam do its work. If you get too hot, open the towel and take a breath of fresh air before going under the towel again. Try to stay in the steam for about five minutes.

Use the steam treatments for rejuvenating mature skin, on acne skin or tired skin. The steam will improve the skin tone as well as the texture of the skin.

You should always end the treatment by splashing cold water onto the skin. Alternatively, you can use ice to massage the skin for perfect tonal balance. Tip: use a plastic popsicle mold to make a massage ice stick by freezing distilled or spring water.) When using ice, massage in upward motions while applying gentle pressure. Remember to never rub the skin dry, rather pat the skin dry with a clean towel.

Steam recipe for normal skin

- 2 drops of Fennel Essential Oil

- 2 drops of Lemon Essential Oil

- 2 drops of Lavender Essential Oil
- 2 drops of Neroli Essential Oil

Mix these essential oils well in a small brown bottle. Use 2 drops of this mix on the water for your steam treatment.

Steam recipe for dry skin

- 2 drops of Chamomile German Essential Oil
- 2 drops of Rose Essential Oil
- 2 drops of Palma Rose Essential Oil
- 2 drops of Bois de Rose Essential Oil

Mix these essential oils well in a small brown bottle. Use 2 drops of this mix on the water for your steam treatment.

Steam recipe for acne

- 2 drops of Clary Sage Essential Oil
- 2 drops of Thyme Essential Oil
- 2 drops of Lavender Essential Oil
- 2 drops of Chamomile Essential Oil

Mix these essential oils well in a small brown bottle. Use 2 drops of this mix on the water for your steam treatment.

Steam recipe for dermatitis

- 2 drops of Clary Sage Essential Oil
- 2 drops of Thyme Essential Oil

- 2 drops of Juniper Essential Oil

- 2 drops of Grapefruit Essential Oil

Mix these essential oils well in a small brown bottle. Use 2 drops of this mix on the water for your steam treatment.

Facial oil recipes

Essential oils greatly enhance the beauty and glow of skin on the face. It can balance normal skin, nourish dry skin, and even treat oily skin.

Moisturizer for normal skin recipe

- 15 drops of Rose Essential Oil

- 5 drops of Chamomile Essential Oil

- 5 drops of Lavender Essential Oil

- 5 drops of Lemon Essential Oil

Dilute all the essential oils in 30 ml of hazelnut oil. Damp your skin and massage the moisturizer onto the face. Lightly tap your face with tissue to remove the excess oil.

Night care recipe for normal skin

- 5 drops of Fennel Essential Oil

- 5 drops of Lemon Essential Oil

- 10 drops of Palma Rosa Essential Oil

- 10 drops of Geranium Essential Oil

Prepare a base oil by adding 10 drops of Evening Primrose essential oil to 30 ml apricot kernel oil. Add the essential oils to this base. Apply on the skin and remove the excess with a tissue.

Moisturizing oil for dry skin recipe

- 15 drops of Chamomile Essential Oil
- 5 drops of Hyssop Essential Oil
- 5 drops of Bois de Rose Essential Oil
- 5 drops of Sandalwood Essential Oil

Prepare a base oil by combining 30 ml of coconut oil with 10 drops of Evening Primrose oil and two drops of Carrot Oil. Mix the essential oils into this base oil. Use this preparation as you would any other moisturizing cream.

Night care recipe for dry skin
For the base oil:

- 10 ml Soya Bean Oil
- 10 ml Avocado Oil
- 10 ml wheat germ oil
- 30 drops Jojoba Oil
- 10 drops Borage Seed Oil
- 20 drops Evening Primrose Oil

Essential oil ingredients:

- 10 drops of Carrot Essential Oil
- 5 drops of Hyssop Essential Oil

- 10 drops of Benzoin Essential Oil

- 15 drops of Geranium Essential Oil

- 10 drops of Chamomile Essential Oil

- 5 drops of Rosemary Essential Oil

First mix all the ingredients for the base oil together. Now add all the essential oil ingredients. Use a small amount of this mixture on the face and dab the excess away with a tissue.

Balancing oil for oily skin recipe

- 2 drops of Rosemary Essential Oil

- 10 drops of Lemon Essential Oil

- 8 drops of Juniper Essential Oil

- 10 drops of Geranium Essential Oil

Prepare a base oil by combining 30 ml of hazelnut oil with 10 drops of carrot oil. Mix the essential oils into this base oil. Gently massage the oil onto the face. Remove the excess by dabbing the face with a tissue.

Night care recipe for dry skin

- 10 drops of Juniper Essential Oil

- 15 drops of Pettigraine Essential Oil

- 5 drops of Marjoram Essential Oil

- 5 drops of Frankincense Essential Oil

- 10 drops of Lemon Essential Oil

Prepare a base oil by adding 10 drops of carrot oil to 30 ml apricot kernel oil. Add all the essential oils to this base. Apply a small amount of this mix to the skin and remove the excess with a tissue.

Away with Wrinkles

We get older every second of every day. The skin ages with us and, over time, it loses the ability to properly regenerate. By using the following recipes, you can combat wrinkles before they become a problem. As we get older, more wrinkles appear and the consistency of the skin changes with time, so the recipes are divided into four age groups.

Over Twenty Wrinkle Recipe

- 1 drop of Carrot Oil

- 3 drops of Chamomile Essential Oil

- 5 drops of Fennel Essential Oil

- 5 drops of Lavender Essential Oil

- 8 drops of Neroli Essential Oil

- 8 drops of Geranium Essential Oil

Dilute these essential oils in the 30 ml of apricot kernel, almond or hazelnut oil.

Over Thirty Wrinkle Recipe

- 2 drops of Patchouli Essential Oil

- 5 drops of Jojoba Essential Oil

- 5 drops of Borage Seed Essential Oil

27

- 5 drops of Carrot Essential Oil

- 7 drops of Fennel Essential Oil

- 8 drops of Rose Essential Oil

- 8 drops of Clary Sage Essential Oil

- 10 drops of Palma Rosa Essential Oil

- 10 drops of Yarrow Essential Oil

Dilute these essential oils in the 30 ml of apricot kernel or hazelnut oil.

Over Forty Wrinkle Recipe

- 2 drops of Rosemary Essential Oil

- 3 drops of Lemon Essential Oil

- 10 drops of Evening Primrose Essential Oil

- 10 drops of Carrot Essential Oil

- 10 drops of Fennel Essential Oil

- 10 drops of Frankincense Essential Oil

- 10 drops of Lavender Essential Oil

- 10 drops of Neroli Essential Oil

Dilute these essential oils in the 30 ml of apricot kernel or hazelnut oil.

Over Fifty Wrinkle Recipe

- 2 drops of Myrrh Essential Oil

- 3 drops of Lavender Essential Oil

- 5 drops of Rose Essential Oil

- 5 drops of Galbanum Essential Oil

- 5 drops of Violet leaf Essential Oil

- 10 drops of Evening Primrose Essential Oil

- 10 drops of Carrot Essential Oil

- 10 drops of Bois de Rose Essential Oil

- 10 drops of Frankincense Essential Oil

- 10 drops of Neroli Essential Oil

Dilute these essential oils in the 30 ml of apricot kernel or hazelnut oil.

Conclusion

Take charge of your health, be natural, and live green. Science is becoming more aware that essential oils, used thousands of years ago, do have a place in contemporary life. Some medical communities may still somewhat skeptical that essential oils can be used in sufficient quantities to have any real curing power, yet, it is proven that essential oils can move through the skin into the bloodstream quickly and with remarkable calming, stimulating or healing properties. The essence crosses the brain-blood barrier and move to all areas of the brain to decrease stress, increase stimulation, and provide emotional feelings of well-being.

Essential oils may not be able to cure diseases, but they do provide physical and emotional support that enhances the body's ability to fight diseases. Essential oils have also been known to delay the onset of disease symptoms.

Aromatherapy is the alternative medicine that sprang up because of essential oils. Aromatherapy brings in the therapeutic use of essential oils for improvement of physical, emotional and spiritual well-being.

Suffice it to say, there are lots of things you can do with essential oils, for the home, for your health, for beauty, and so much more. Make a natural sunscreen, eliminate soap scum from the shower curtain, clean burn pans, cleanse air in smelly homes, clean and refresh carpets, keep pests away, and eliminate mold. Natural essential oils can be used to reduce stress and anxiety, invigorate the mind, focus, to increase the level of spiritual enlightenment, relieve tension, whiten your teeth, treat burns, reduce the seriousness of sinusitis, remove wrinkles, detoxify your body, and even to purify your fridge. Even those smelly shoes can be a thing of the past, courtesy of natural essential oils, and the recipes for all of these purposes need not cost a lot.

The uses for essential oils are potentially endless. Essential oils are a natural and fun way to improve your surroundings, wherever you are, and an easy way to promote your health and well-being, both mentally and physically.